The Human Resources Agenda

An action checklist

Roy C. Lilley
Chairman
Homewood NHS Trust

and

Chris Wilson
Director of Human Resources
Homewood NHS Trust

Foreword by
Eric Caines
Director of Health Services Management
Nottingham University

RADCLIFFE MEDICAL PRESS • OXFORD AND NEW YORK

©1994 Radcliffe Medical Press Ltd.
15 Kings Meadow, Ferry Hinksey Road, Oxford OX2 0DP

141 Fifth Avenue, New York, NY 10010, USA

British Library Cataloguing in Publication Data
A catalogue record for this book is available from the British Library.

ISBN 1 85775 077 2

Typeset by AMA Graphics Ltd, Preston
Printed and bound in Great Britain by
Biddles Ltd, Guildford and King's Lynn

. . . for everyone who lives in the shadow of Eric.

---

*The only limit to an organization is the
imagination of the people it employs*

Bill Gates, Chairman, Microsoft

Bill Gates is right. Imagination is the only limiting factor to the success of any enterprise. It is the vision of the people in the organization which makes the organization what it is. The enthusiasm of the employees can carry an organization through bad times; commitment from staff can be the difference between success and failure.

The fashion for putting organizational methodology under the microscope is probably past. Today the focus is on developing people. No matter how well the enterprise is structured, badly trained, demoralized staff will never make an organization successful.

Commitment, enthusiasm and self-belief from the men and women who come to work every day are the starting point for change and the turning point for developing the future.

Roy Lilley
Chris Wilson

Contents

Foreword xi

Introduction 1

How to make this book work for you 2

Section 1: Corporate shaping 3

Action Check 1: Organizational values 5

Action Check 2: Business strategy 7

Action Check 3: Culture 10

Action Check 4 : HR delivery 12

Section 2: Re-engineering the HR agenda 13

Action Check 5: The Board and pay 15

Action Check 6: Using Trust freedoms 16

Action Check 7: Commitment of managers 17

Action Check 8:   Teamworking   19

Action Check 9:   Pay – researching alternatives   23

Action Check 10:   Recognition   25

Action Check 11:   Pay – Does the organization have   31
                   access to pay modelling?

Action Check 12:   Pay – Does the organization   33
                   understand its workforce?

Action Check 13:   Pay – What are the design factors to   36
                   take into account when remodelling
                   pay?

Action Check 14:   Pay – Is a 'pay spine' to be used?   41
                   How will it be designed?

Action Check 15:   Pay - Will pay be linked to   47
                   performance?

Action Check 16:   Pay - Will redesigned pay include an   49
                   annual uplift?

Action Check 17:   Pay - What are the dangers of   50
                   introducing a new scheme?

Action Check 18:   Pay – Is overtime a concern?   51

Action Check 19:   Sickness   53

Action Check 20:   Non-pay issues   56

Action Check 21:   Payroll   58

Action Check 22:   The workforce – What arc thc bcncfits   61
                   of reprofiling?

Action Check 23:   The workforce – Can jobs be   63
                   redesigned around the needs of the
                   organization?

Action Check 24:   Performance management – Can   66
                   individual performance be improved?

Action Check 25 : Performance management – How   70
                   does performance management work?

Action Check 26 : Performance management – How will   73
                   productivity issues be handled?

Action Check 27:   Training – What is the role of training   75
                   in the organization?

Action Check 28:   Training – Can training needs be met   78
                   in house?

Action Check 29 : Training and management – How will   80
                   the process of re-engineering be
                   managed?

Action Check 30:   Training and management – What are   81
                   the effects of restructuring on HR?

Action Check 31:   Training and management – How will   83
                   skills be developed?

Action Check 32:   Training and management – How are   86
                   managers developed?

Action Check 33: Manpower information   88

Action Check 34: Induction   90

Action Check 35: Recruitment   93

Action Check 36: Retention   95

Action Check 37: Discipline   98

Action Check 38: Equal opportunities   102

Action Check 39: Employing women   104

Action Check 40: AIDS and HIV   108

Action Check 41: Hepatitis B   111

Section 3: Measuring success   113

Action Check 42: Success   115

Index   119

Foreword

If ever there was a time for action in the human resource (HR) field in the NHS – for doing things as opposed to talking about doing them or talking about what needs to be done – it has to be now. The challenges for the HR function have never been greater than they are at present. This book sets out the agenda with such unequivocal clarity and tight logic that there can be no excuse, at the very least, for not making a start on the fundamental process of reshaping how work should be done and how to reward those who do it.

The appeal of the book is its straightforward commonsense. Without using fancy language it speaks directly not only to the HR professional but also to the Chief Executive, Chairman or other Board directors who want to have a feel for what their personnel department ought to be doing. Its timing is ideal and it should have a great impact.

ERIC CAINES
Director of Health Services Management
Nottingham University
February 1994

Introduction

The NHS is going through a time of great change. Nowhere is that change felt more than in the human resource (HR) profession.

The management of change, delivery of new services, training and a reshaping of old attitudes falls to the HR team to lead and deliver. All NHS Trusts are facing a revolution. In the last ten years a revolution in medical technology has reduced average bed stays from ten days to just over six. That figure is set to halve in the next five years. Some predict that, by the year 2000, more than half of all procedures could be day cases. What this means for a Trust cannot be underestimated. The pressure will be for fewer and fewer hospitals of the type we know today. We will see a shift to primary care, away from old style hospitals and into a new world delivered by medical technology in a spiral of development and change.

New thinking about what that means for jobs, how organizations are engineered and how services are delivered will be at the top of the list for NHS Trust Boards and HR professionals.

Old style pay bargaining must give way to performance management and organizations will look to the HR team to develop ways of using pay and rewards as a stepping stone to greater productivity.

This book examines some of the issues raised by this change. It does not presume to have the answers. It is a signpost for issues and a foundation for thinking and brainstorming. It allows the reader to come to their own conclusions about the relevance of the issues and think about how to devise answers appropriate to the needs of their situation.

How to make this book work for you

This book is not the work of authors who claim to have all the answers. It has been written by two people who have experience in succeeding (and occasionally failing!) with human resource (HR) policies and radical approaches. Their experience has come from asking themselves questions about how to take the next step.

It aims to raise issues. Issues which, sooner or later, will be important to every NHS Trust. The issues become questions, questions which your organization may be seeking to answer.

In this book the issues are the Action Checks. They are summarized, helping to shape thinking around key points. Flowing from the Action Checks is a cluster of questions. The questions provide the thinking points. Points for the Board to consider and for the HR team to address.

Use the book as an aid to brainstorming; as a help to developing policy; as a checklist; a crib sheet and an aide memoire. Some of the questions are answers in themselves.

Think of the book as a map, plotting the path to policy development and delivery.

SECTION 1

CORPORATE SHAPING

Action Check 1

Organizational values

Does the organization publish a set of values and have a clear mission?

A clear Mission and Values statement will be the starting point for much of the work of the Board. Properly thought through they will be the bedrock on which to build, the standard against which the organization will measure itself and the signpost for the future.

Included in those values should be a commitment to the staff, their conditions and development. Each organization will approach the matter in its own way but should consider including the following points.

o The organization values all its staff, wherever they make their contribution; they will be encouraged and empowered in their work, treated fairly, offered equal opportunity to develop and be listened to, carefully.

o It is from this statement that all HR policy should flow; translating the philosophy into a practical operational agenda.

o Value statements must be owned by the whole organization and not only the Board. If everyone is going to be able to have their say in drafting the Mission and Values statement, it will take care and time.

- Who will take the lead in drafting the document?

- How will everyone be given the chance to make a con-tribution?

- How will the views be evaluated and incorporated into the final document?

- Will staff whose first language is not English be given the chance to take part and will the results be published in their language?

Action Check 2

Business strategy

Does the organization have clear and deliverable Business and Strategic goals?

The business plan forms the basis for the year's activity and the strategic plan the foundation for the future. The NHS is operating in a period of great change. No NHS Trust is immune from the effects of change. Merging, downsizing and service reprofiling are the language of tomorrow. Careful and accurate sensitivity analysis of the threats and opportunities to specialties and services is vital.

The development of the business and strategic plan will take time and should be a document with which the whole organization is comfortable. Senior HR practitioners should be involved from the beginning and the impact of the business plan on the HR function will need scrupulous evaluation. If a great deal of change is planned, the HR team must be involved at the outset, to ensure that they are able to prepare the staff for what is ahead. For example, new ventures may be identified for the future, in which case training and other development needs must be evaluated and planned.

♦ Does the Board know what the options are?

◆ Has the Board reviewed the options?

◆ Has the Board arrived at a clear view of what it wants?

◆ Has it shared those ideas with the rest of the organization?

◆ Is the Board looking to the HR director for inspiration?

◆ Has the HR team been fully involved in the business planning process?

◆ Has the impact of changes been thoroughly assessed?

◆ Does the HR team know what is expected of them? Are they prepared and resourced?

◆ Strategic planning is generally long range and it is here that structural changes in service delivery may be identified. Has the HR team had an input to the long range strategic plan and been able to assess the 'people' consequences of it?

Action Check 3

Culture

Is everyone in the organization enthusiastic about the idea of Trusts and their freedoms? Attitude surveys can provide some of the answers. How highly is pay rated as a concern among staff? Everyone would probably like to have more money but surveys undertaken in the NHS indicate that pay is not always at the top of the agenda for health service staff. People working in patient care areas of the NHS will have a commitment to a client group and often will wish to see more resources available for patients. Sometimes education and training increase enthusiasm more than simple cash rewards. A locally based pay strategy can address these issues and provide a meaningful policy approach that may not be based on pay alone. Study leave, training to use new equipment and staff development may all have a part to play.

♦ What is the organization's 'go-button' and how can it be pressed? What makes the staff enthusiastic and is it the same for all of them or does it vary from department to department, and staff group to staff group?

- ◆ Can an attitude questionnaire be devised in house?

- ◆ How will the results be evaluated?

- ◆ Will everyone in the organization see the results?

- ◆ Can the results be interpreted into new policies?

- ◆ How often should this exercise be repeated?

Action Check 4

HR delivery

The HR agenda is probably the most important of all the foundation strategies in an NHS Trust. In a typical Trust something
between 70 and 80 percent of the revenue budget, derived from
contract income, is spent on staff and most of the services are,
in industry terms, labour intensive. The question is, how to make
the wage and salary bill an investment and a stepping stone to
better performance and efficiency and not a millstone, dragging
the organization backwards, into the past?

HR management is about the key to the future. HR strategies
can be tailored to deliver the status quo, gradual change or swift
remodelling. What is required?

It is possible to devise an HR strategy that places pay at the
fulcrum point of higher rewards and better performance. HR
strategies can deal with the management of change, poor morale
and lack of commitment from staff. A good HR approach can
also deliver performance management, training, staff recruitment
and retention and address unacceptable levels of sickness and
absence.

The trick to having HR strategies that work is to have a clear
understanding of what you want them to deliver, how they are
going to deliver and who is accountable for their delivery. In
particular, the Board must have a clear idea about what it wants
the HR service to deliver and what success will look like.

SECTION 2

RE-ENGINEERING THE HR AGENDA

Action Check 5

The Board and pay

Does the Board wish to introduce a local pay and reward strategy?

There are very few industries which would be happy for the rates of pay of their staff to be decided by third parties from outside their own organizations. Keeping control of the wages and salaries bill seems like sensible management. There may be a number of reasons why the Board wish to move away from centrally negotiated pay bargaining and deal with the entire matter in-house.

Apart from wanting to exercise control over costs, there may be reasons, relating to performance management, why the Board wishes to see change take place. The Board may wish to find ways of rewarding staff who perform well and incentivize those who do not. Local pay arrangements can be the foundation for perform-ance management. Whatever the reasons, the Board must think through its strategy; decide what it wishes to achieve and how to go about it.

More fundamentally, the HR team must have a clear decision from the Board, complete support and an unambiguous mandate.

Action Check 6

Using Trust freedoms

A local pay strategy?

Enshrined in the legislation which permits Health Service Units to become NHS Trusts, (The NHS and Community Care Act 1990), is the freedom for Trusts to establish their own pay and reward strategies. This should be the big challenge for HR professionals and the opportunity to deliver real change. However, few Trusts have taken advantage of that freedom. Why? Trusts which have taken the big step of creating their own, local, pay and benefits arrangements report great gains for their organizations.

Nevertheless, the complexities of the task should not be underestimated. The transition requires thorough planning, the total commitment of the Board and the confidence of staff that they are not going to be worse off!

Action Check 7

Commitment of managers

Are senior managers committed to a local pay strategy?

What is the involvement and commitment of key players in the design and implementation of the plan? Assuming the Board is fully committed to the policy, what about the senior managers? A local pay strategy may mean realignment of departmental budgets. Are managers prepared for that?

♦ Are senior managers committed to the scheme?

♦ Do they really know what it might mean for them, their budgets and their staff?

♦ How will the results be evaluated?

◆ Will everyone in the organization see the results?

◆ Can the results be interpreted into new policies?

Action Check 8

Teamworking

Can the Executive Team work together?

Making the change from centrally negotiated pay bargaining to local strategies is not just a task for the HR department. As well as the implications for staff and their representatives, there are serious financial considerations. The development of the scheme must be a joint project for the finance department and the HR team. For such a complex and sensitive task to be completed successfully they must share the same understanding of the purpose of the job in hand. For example, if the HR team wishes to influence staff retention difficulties, it is no good if the finance department believes the purpose is to cut staff numbers.

- ◆ Is there a shared understanding of purpose between the departments?

- ◆ Has careful consideration been given to what you want to influence and the outcomes that will be sought?

- What is the culture of the departments involved? How does it differ from department to department?

- Perceptions may differ between levels of the hierarchy within departments. Is any departmental cultural change necessary before the main work can be put in hand?

- Do the finance and HR teams work well together?

- Who will take the lead in the process?

- The focus should be on a single leader; one accountable person who has clear authority to act and who reports directly to the Board. Who is that person?

◆ Do you have the necessary depth within your HR and finance functions to deliver a policy with the complexity of a local pay strategy?

◆ How are the executive directors rewarded?

◆ Are the executive directors rewarded individually or as a team?

◆ Can executive directors rewards be linked to the performance of the Board in total?

◆ Pay budgets may have to be 'unpicked' and funds reallo-
cated. Sensitive negotiations with budget-holders will be
required and possible discussions with staffside representatives will all require skill, tact and experience. Can
the organization deliver a major policy shift at this time?

Action Check 9

Pay – researching alternatives

What are the alternatives to 'Whitley'?

To replace the 'Whitley' pay scales and not merely replicate them locally, someone in the organization must have a good knowledge of the technical structure of the 'Whitley' pay scales, how they operate and what the strengths and weaknesses of the system are. It may also be helpful to look at a range of other organizations, both inside and outside of the public sector, to see how they pay their staff. This will help in developing an under-standing of how pay systems are constructed and their effect.

♦ Who has the necessary knowledge?

♦ If it is not 'in-house', how will it be acquired?

♦ Which other organizations could you look at?

Action Check 10

Recognition

Will the organization recognize trade unions?

There is no obligation on an NHS Trust to recognize trade unions or staff organizations. However, good staff relations policies dictate that serious consideration should be given to the whole issue of staff representation. Measured nationally, trade union membership is falling and there is as much of an issue about how to hold a dialogue with non-trade union members as there is about formal arrangements to talk with trade unions. The introduction of local pay and reward strategies, where annual pay is negotiated locally, can cause quite a headache for some staff-side bodies as well as some local managers. For many unions and staff organizations, national pay agreements mean negotiations are undertaken, by full-time officers, at a national level and local representatives have little experience in dealing with the complexities of pay. Before the introduction of local pay bargaining, local trade unionists may need some reassurance; they may wish to involve the full-time, union officer in discussions.

♦ Will it be better to recognize staff-side groups before or after any new pay strategy is in place, or should recognition be part of the 'new deal'?

◆ Is it necessary for trade unions to be recognized for local pay bargaining to be implemented?

◆ Are trade unions already recognized and what are the terms of recognition?

◆ If the answer is no, should trade unions be recognized locally and on what terms?

◆ If there is more than one union/professional organization, will all of them be recognized?

♦ Might it be possible, if there are a number of unions seeking recognition, to recognize them all, but only negotiate with a fixed number at any one time at a single table, leaving the unions to decide amongst themselves who should attend meetings?

♦ What is the relationship between the design of the pay bargaining machinery and the design of the local pay structure?

♦ What is the relationship between a single table bargaining set-up and the design of your local pay structure?

♦ Is multiple table bargaining an option? Meetings with separate staff-side groups and organizations separately? What are the implications for time and confusion?

- If the local trade unionists are inexperienced, will the organization assist in their training, either by giving 'time-out' to attend training or by providing training opportunities?

- In what forum will meetings and discussions take place? How many staff-side representatives and how many from the management side?

- Will any non-executive directors take part in the process?

- Who will chair the meetings? Will it be more productive and less confrontational if the Chair is shared or rotated?

♦ Will the full-time union officials have a role in the meeting forum or will it be better if they attend as observers?

♦ Is the organization prepared to share detailed financial and operational information with the staffside? Particularly in relation to pay and other financial claims? Is it likely to support management's case, if there is an open book approach?

♦ If expectations are not met by the arrangements, how will disagreements be settled and an agreement be changed or terminated?

♦ In the event of a disagreement, will there be a facility for conciliation and arbitration?

+ What are the types of arbitration for the organization to consider? Standard arbitration seeks to find a solution based on consent and a willingness to find middle ground – this can be costly and time consuming for both sides. Pendulum arbitration seeks to find for one side only. What are the implications of these different approaches for your organization?

+ What about those staff not in a trade union? How will their voice be heard? Will they have a place at the meeting table, alongside trade unionists? Should management insist upon it? How will non-unionists choose their representatives? How long will they stand for?

+ Will you seek to make any agreement legally binding?

Action Check 11

Pay – Does the organization have access to pay modelling?

Access to an accurate pay modelling facility is vital. A proper breakdown of what staff currently earn, plus all other emoluments and benefits is not always easy to obtain. Not until the current pay situation has been understood will it be possible to offer meaningful alternatives. What information do you need?

♦ Is the information available? Where from?

♦ Will it take time to obtain?

◆ Some NHS payroll data is famous for being inaccurate! Is the information that is being sought accurate and what is the test of accuracy?

Action Check 12

Pay – Does the organization understand its workforce?

Does the HR department have a detailed knowledge of the workforce? Understanding the character of the workforce and what influences it is important. A range of issues may have a bearing on its performance and costs.

♦ The difference between establishment staff numbers and wholetime equivalents can have a huge impact on payroll costs. What are the implications?

♦ Is there a high turnover of staff? Is it related to particular work areas, skills or age groups? High staff turnover means high recruitment costs and high costs for covering absences. Are there areas of stability? What conclusions may be drawn?

- What is the age profile of the organization? Are there likely to be a number of retirements coming up all together? Is this good news or bad?

- What are sickness levels like? Is longterm sickness a problem? Is short term sickness 'the real thing' or is it used as an excuse for a day off?

- Are there problems in recruiting in certain skill groups? What are the solutions?

- What is the status of the job market outside the organization? Are there local skill shortages that impact on the organization? Are there skills that could be used, retrained or encouraged to work in the organization?

♦ How flexible are the organization's employment con-
    tracts? What is the breakdown between full and part-time
    staff? How common is job sharing?

Action Check 13

Pay – What are the design factors to take into account when remodelling pay?

Opportunity for carrying out major overhauls of pay and reward approaches does not often arise. When the opportunity presents itself it is important that the maximum possible benefit is taken. The extent to which pay design can reflect skill mix and any staff reprofiling changes you may wish to make is significant. Job evaluation of all posts before designing a new system is highly desirable. The choice of evaluation system comes into question as do issues of timing and speed. The process should be undertaken by someone with knowledge of the service but not operationally involved with the day-to-day operations. This does not necessarily mean external consultants from the private sector. Might it be possible to arrive at an arrangement with an adjoining Trust with similar ambitions, and work together? If the answer is yes, what system could you use? Does it matter if you do this before or after the pay design or implementation stage?

The position of staff coming into Trust status is protected in law. The Transfer of Undertaking (Protection of Employment) Regulations covers the status and working conditions of staff. There is no obligation on them to agree to new conditions of service. How will you attract them to the new pay spine?

♦ Is it necessary to introduce job evaluation? Should it be for all posts or just for some? What is the rationale behind the decision?

♦ Should job evaluation be based on the existing 'Whitley' stereotype or on a new, reprofiled, redesigned job – or both?

♦ Should job evaluation be introduced as a preliminary to a new pay strategy or can it be left until later?

♦ Who will carry out the evaluations? Is there anyone appropriately qualified in the organization?

♦ Should the job evaluation system be approved by trade unions?

♦ Should the evaluation system be developed specifically for the NHS or could it be taken from industry or commerce? Could the system be designed in-house?

♦ What kind of job evaluation system best suits the organization's needs?

♦ Should the approach be: ranking/grading, job classification, factor comparison, a points system or a combination of them all?

♦ What are the cost implications?

♦ Can a strategy be introduced without 'new' money?

♦ Can other directorates be persuaded to contribute savings or cash to make money available to pump-prime a new pay initiative?

♦ Can savings in the organization be dedicated to getting a new pay initiative off the ground?

♦ Can the costs of overtime and agency nursing be limited, to produce savings to get a local initiative under way?

♦ Will the outcome of the evaluation process be used as a basis for the design of new pay procedures?

- 'Whitley' is composed of a number of complex 'pay spines'. They lead to inequalities and complexity. If a new strategy is to be based on pay spines; how many pay spines are practicable or feasible? Can the aim be to get to one spine for the whole organization?

- Under 'Whitley', progression up the pay spine is on an incremental points basis; what size are the new spine point differentials going to be? The number of spine points and the margins between them could have a major impact on the length of the spine and, more significantly, on the costs. Check the full year effect of the proposed spine over several years, taking into account the staff profile, turnover and their grades and seniority.

- How will staff progress up the spine? Progress could be by performance of the individual, performance of the team or by length of service. Indeed, progress could be by a combination of all three. If the new policy is to deliver organizational goals, on which of the three should the most emphasis be placed?

Action Check 14

Pay – Is a 'pay spine' to be used? How will it be designed?

Pay spines can have bands, in effect grouping staff together in one segment on the spine. Transferring from existing pay arrangements to the new means assessing the point (or band) at which the transfer is made. Progress from one band to another, or movement between the bands, can depend on long service or improved competence. Will you include bandings on the pay spine?

If yes, how many should there be and how should they relate to each other? They could overlap or butt up to each other? Transition from one band to another will increase costs. What will trigger transition from one band to another, and what are the rules for joining the spine at a particular band?

♦ How will staff join the spine? Will it depend on job evaluation?

- What happens when staff get to the top of their banding? Will they remain there or automatically move up to the next band? Will they still have access to performance related pay (if it applies to them)?

- Is there lateral movement within bands to allow for performance rewards without moving up to the next band?

- Is there a presumption that all movement will be upwards, or could poor performance result in movement down the spine?

Pay spine – Example 1

15 10696
14 10384
13 10082
12   9788
11   9503
10   9226
 9   8957
 8   8696
 7   8443
 6   8197
 5   7958
 4   7726
 3   7501
 2   7283
 1   7071

This is an example of a straightforward pay spine. It can be designed to feature both constant and inconsistent differentials between each band. The location of jobs at an appropriate place on the spine (ie 'spot salaries') depends on existing pay, and the results would normally take account of a job evaluation exercise. Performance pay increments can be paid within bands without advancing up the spine. For example, a performance increment of around £200 can be paid within spine band one and spine band two and so on.

Pay spine – Example 2

		13 10082
		12 9788
		11 9503
		10 9226
		9 8957
9	8957	Band three
8	8696	
7	8443	
6	8197	
5	7958	

5	7958	Band two
4	7726	
3	7501	
2	7283	
1	7071	

Band one

This typical 'Whitley' style structure contains jobs within pay bands (or grades). The top of Band one is the bottom of Band two and so on. This approach is useful where differences between jobs are marginal.

Pay spine – Example 3

		5	9503
		4	9226
		3	8957
		2	8696
5	7958	1	8443
4	7726	Band two	
3	7501		
2	7283		
1	7071		
Band one			

This example shows a large gap between each grade. It can be used when there are significant differences between types of work undertaken by a group (or groups) of staff.

Pay spine – Example 4

```
                        14 10679
                        13 10171
                        12  9687
        10  9226        11  9226
         9  8957         Band two
         8  8696
         7  8443
         6  8197
         5  7958
         4  7726
         3  7501
         2  7283
         1  7071
        Band one
```

This example illustrates band size and varying differentials. It is designed to reflect differences in responsibility, job size or other features.

Action Check 15

Pay – Will pay be linked to performance?

Performance pay can be a powerful tool for the organization to use as a lever for better performance and quality. Will the Board agree to set aside a particular amount of money for performance pay and rewards? Will the amount be linked to the overall performance of the organization? How will it be determined? Will it be 'ringfenced' and impossible to vier to other parts of the budget?

♦ How is performance pay to be paid? At the end of the year when performance is assessed and agreed, or as an 'allowance' against anticipated performance, but with a claw back agreement in the event of under performance? Can there be a quarterly assessment where some recognition of performance can be made?

♦ Will performance pay be consolidated into normal pay or paid as a separate, visible bonus? When will it be paid?

♦ How will staff be assimilated into the new arrangements? Is there scope to consolidate some current fixed allowances such as London Weighting, Nursing Leads etc.?

♦ What links will there be with the performance management process? Will pay be used as an incentive to better performance?

Action Check 16

Pay – Will redesigned pay include an annual uplift?

In the past, annual uplifts in pay have been fiercely fought over. Indeed some unions have felt so strongly that industrial action has been contemplated and, in extreme cases, taken. Is there a right to a regular annual increase or should all increases be earned and result from increased performance?

♦ How will the expectation of annual increases be addressed? Is there a need to keep in step with the 'Whitley' scale? Does an annual uplift automatically apply to all staff groups?

♦ If increases are to be based on other factors, how much information does the organization have about the local labour market? Who are the organization's competitors and how much do they pay their employees?

Action Check 17

Pay – What are the dangers of introducing a new scheme?

All new schemes can bring drawbacks as well as benefits. It is important to be aware of some of the problems which may result from the introduction of a local pay and reward strategy.

Look out for escalating pay costs if you get it wrong! If people come into the scheme at too high a level, costs can get out of control. Similarly, if performance targets are set too low, the wages and salary costs will rocket up, as staff perform indifferently and benefit from too high a reward.

Make sure the new scheme does not simply recreate a 'local Whitley scale'. 'Whitley' is complex and will not leave room for performance pay to be raised as appropriate in individual cases.

Does the organization have good pay information systems? Keeping in touch with the market is fundamentally important. Watching the local press, maintaining a pay database and networking with other HR professionals may provide the answer.

At first trade unions may be nervous about the new package. However, once they become accustomed to it, what will this mean for the organization. Are strong unions beneficial or not?

How will managers react? Managers must be committed to performance management. They are likely to need significant extra training which requires time and money.

How will doctors be involved in the process? What is the impact and future of merit awards?

Action Check 18

Pay – Is overtime a concern?

How much overtime does the organization work? Is it good value for money or does it need to be reduced? Similarly, agency nurses cost about 30 percent more than those employed directly. Why does the organization need to employ them? Can voids in shifts be filled by Bank staff?

- ◆ What is the cost of overtime? Could that money be better used by increasing the staff of the organization? Can voids and absences be covered by an internal bank arrangement?

- ◆ Can an internal bank arrangement be negotiated to allow greater flexibility and reduce running costs?

♦ What are bank rates of pay likely to be? Will they be attractive enough for staff to want to work for them? Will the staff side organizations agree?

♦ Are medical locum costs examined regularly?

Action Check 19

Sickness

What is the organization's sick record? What is the cost to the organization? Anything over four per cent is above industry white and blue collar norms. Is sickness managed?

Can a formula be applied to sickness absences?

What does this formula reveal about evaluating sickness records?

$S \times S \times D$

Where S = the number of spells of absence in the last 52 weeks and D = the number of days of absence in the last 52 weeks

So, for example, three employees with 12 days' absence in one year, but differently distributed, can produce dramatically different scores: one absence of 12 days = 12 points; six absences of two days = 432 points; 12 absences of 1 day = 1728 points.

◆ What other methods can be used to highlight repeated episodes of short term sickness and their relationship to days off differentiating between real sickness and absenteeism?

♦ What is the role of the occupational health service? What is expected of it? Do they see themselves as service providers or independent practitioners?

♦ Will managers be expected to make welfare visits, to check on the progress of staff who have reported sick?

♦ Will there be an attempt to separate long term sickness from short episodes of repeated sickness?

♦ Should sickness league tables be published?

♦ Will persistent sick leave takers be informally warned about their conduct? Will formal disciplinary action be taken against those whose sickness record is poor and in doubt?

♦ Will all absences through sickness require a medical certificate?

♦ Will staff returning from sick leave be required to review their state of health with the occupational health service?

♦ Who is responsible to the Board for improving the sickness record of the organization?

Action Check 20

Non-pay issues

Is there more to reward than pay?

Restructuring the organization's pay and reward policies should include a range of non-pay issues. There are a range of options which are worth looking at.

♦ Reductions or increases in the hours worked are not without cost but can be worth consideration. Is it worthwhile considering standardizing the working week, for all staff? What is the likely staff reaction?

♦ How does annual leave fit into the equation? Is there benefit in bringing entitlements into line? What are the cost implications and are they manageable?

♦ Shift and night duty payments could also be brought into line. Simpler accounting for pay roll may have some cash saving dividends. Is it a viable option?

♦ Weekend and bank holiday rates could also be consolidated. Is this practical or helpful?

♦ Can statutory days be treated in the same way?

Action Check 21

Payroll

How accurate is the payroll?

In a large organization with a great many different pay scales and allowances mistakes can be common. A wage packet or salary slip which is not correct first time costs time and money to put right and is very demotivating for the recipient. A new pay system can exacerbate problems. Does the payroll system have the capacity to cope with your proposed new pay system? Is this a good time to introduce a new, integrated payroll and personnel and manpower system? Can the wages/salary department become a zero defect department?

♦ Is the Board aware of payroll failures? Who is accountable to the Board?

♦ Is data input from managers consistently reliable?

- Who checks the data input for mistakes?

- Who handles payroll and why? Is it done this way because it has always been? When was it last tested?

- What is the cost per entry?

- Has the cost of handling payroll in-house been market tested against the cost of providing the service through an outside firm or bureau?

- What is the cost per correction and who pays for the mistakes?

◆ What is the number of mistakes expressed as a percentage of the whole?

◆ Who apologizes to staff when their salary or wage is incorrectly calculated?

◆ Do the payroll staff understand that they are providing a service? Will they receive customer service training?

Action Check 22

The workforce – What are the benefits of reprofiling?

The reprofiling of jobs, and a review of the skills needed to carry them out successfully, may produce interesting results. Many of the customs and practices acceptable in the past may not be so in the future, particularly if the organization is to undergo radical change. A careful assessment needs to be carried out, to evaluate the current jobs and work practices in the organization; only then can work be undertaken to see how jobs fit into the organization's need, rather than the organization fitting around the jobs!

♦ Is a skill mix review on the HR agenda?

♦ Who will carry out the assessment work? Is there sufficient experience to be able to carry out the work in-house or will outside consultants be required? How will consultants be chosen; for their track record, experience, or some other factors?

♦ The process of review may release cash savings. Will the savings be subsumed into general operational savings, or can they be used in more creative, high profile ways to improve services? Can an understanding of how savings will be employed be agreed before the savings are made and used as an incentive to carry forward change? Does the process recognize that staff are much more likely to co-operate with a savings programme if they can see tangible benefits as a result?

♦ Will a review be opposed by staff-side organizations? Can they be brought in as part of the process? Is it easy to demonstrate benefits to patients or staff, or both?

♦ Will the review create more interesting job opportunities?

♦ How will a review translate into the future? Will the review take into account the local job market, demographics and the needs of the business plan?

Action Check 23

The workforce – Can jobs be redesigned around the needs of the organization?

In a fast changing job market, talented people are placing greater emphasis on job satisfaction. Job design can be a valuable ingredient in the skill mix and reprofiling programme. Developing more relevant and interesting jobs aids staff retention and cuts recruitment costs.

♦ Once skill mix and reprofiling is complete, who will be responsible for ensuring that job design is kept up to date?

♦ Will staff be able to design their own jobs?

- ◆ What impact will technology have on job design?

- ◆ Is job design for the whole organization or can it only be achieved for lower grades and non-medical staff?

- ◆ What are the implications for the medics and other professional groups?

- ◆ What are the implications for working women?

- ◆ What are the implications of these goals on staff skill mix, recruitment and retention?

♦ What are the training implications of skill mix and reprofiling?

Action Check 24

Performance management – Can individual performance be improved?

Gone are the days when staff were paid for turning up! What they achieve and how they perform are now important factors. Performance management need not be about the number of patients treated; it can just as easily be about how patients, their relatives and carers are looked after. Whilst individual performance targets need not be about organizational goals, they must relate to the development of the individual within the organization. Performance managed is an exciting management tool. The performance of individuals can be measured and used to help develop members of staff. Group performance can be measured to encourage teamworking.

♦ Should you aim for a system which is based on individual or team performance, or both?

◆ Who will carry out performance reviews? Are in-house managers able to carry out performance reviews? Are the managers sufficiently highly regarded by the rest of the staff for the results of reviews to go unchallenged, or will in-house staff need training? Does everyone understand that a great deal of initial effort will need to go into training managers in a new system?

◆ Will systems be simple to operate and understood by everyone? Complexity can cause confusion and inconsistency and lead to the appraisal scheme being undermined. Will this trap be avoided?

◆ Is the organization willing to invest the necessary resources not only to introduce the process, but also to maintain and monitor it?

◆ What will be the basis for monitoring, and how will the system be judged? What will the criteria be?

♦ Does the organization recognize a link between pay and performance?

♦ How can you ensure that the organization has the capacity to deliver on important by-products of the process (e.g. non-performance, personal development plans).

♦ How can you ensure that, whenever possible, the emphasis is on measurable, quantifiable performance.

♦ Objectives/goals should be a mix of performance standards/targets, competencies and quality standards/targets, and should aim to maintain and develop the job .

♦ To what extent can you use pay design to reflect skill mix/reprofiling changes which you may wish to make?

Action Check 25

Performance management – How does performance management work?

Performance management is complex and requires high levels of skill and effort to introduce it successfully. Managers who assess performance must be seen as fair and be trusted by the staff they are evaluating. The introduction of performance management can bring lasting benefits, but do not underestimate the size of the task required to carry it out.

♦ Is there a thorough understanding of performance management in the organization?

♦ Does the human resource/personnel/training function have sufficient experience and strength to be able to introduce it without outside help?

♦ Would a scheme apply to the whole organization?

♦ Is it possible or practical to part-start the process?

♦ Will there be staff-side resistance to the introduction of a scheme? How will it be overcome?

♦ Are managers perceived by the rest of the staff as being sufficiently competent to introduce, run and monitor a performance management scheme?

♦ What training needs to be carried out, in advance of the introduction of performance management?

♦ What are the aims of introducing such a scheme?

♦ How will success be measured?

Action Check 26

Performance management – How will productivity issues be handled?

Can productivity be spoken of in the NHS? How will it be measured and by whom? Does productivity mean higher volume of patients or better outcomes for patients, or both? How do staff costs fit into the equation? As contracts with purchasers become more demanding and there is a greater requirement for value for money, productivity issues will take on a greater significance. Can unit labour costs be calculated?

♦ What does productivity mean to the Board?

♦ What does productivity mean to the rest of the organization?

- Does it mean the same to both parties?

- Can the benefits of higher productivity be translated into benefits for patients and staff?

- Will increases in productivity involve new deals with the clinicians?

- In order to achieve higher productivity will a skill mix review be required?

- Does productivity involve the use of capital assets as well as people assets?

Action Check 27

Training – What is the role of training in the organization?

Training budgets can be vulnerable. If the organization is facing financial difficulties it is often the training budget which is cut first. A commitment to training is likely to be popular and very motivational for staff who attach a high significance to training.

◆ How is training targeted to meet the needs of the organization?

◆ What percentage of the budget is spent on training; how does it compare from year to year?

- Where does the training department fit into the management hierarchy?

- Do managers willingly make staff available to attend training courses, or do operational needs come first?

- What are the ratios between in-house training and training which is purchased externally?

- How are outcomes of training measured?

- When outside conferences and training courses are attended how is the information gained shared with the rest of the organization?

* What controls are there over expenditure on attendance on outside conferences?

Action Check 28

Training – Can training needs be met in-house?

In-house training can be expensive to set up, but provides consistency and an understanding of the organization's needs. Outside consultants bring an independent perspective which can give an edge to training. What will the organization do about training?

♦ Can the training needs of the organization be met from a single source?

♦ Can the whole of the training function be provided out-of-house?

♦ Should it be?

♦ Can an in-house training facility be used as an income generation opportunity, providing training for other NHS Trusts or local industry?

♦ How does the Board get to know about the effectiveness of training?

Action Check 29

Training and management – How will the process of re-engineering be managed?

Re-engineering the processes of management throughout the whole organization is not a fast process. What are the time imperatives for completing the process?

♦ Has the programme been shared with the Board and is there wide ownership of the timescale and its implications throughout the organization?

Action Check 30

Training and management – What are the effects of restructuring on HR?

If the business plan requires new services, restructuring, reprofiling or other changes in staffing, what role will training play and
what are the costs?

♦ How will the training department know what is expected
  of them?

♦ Will the training department have an input into the business plan especially where innovation or reconfiguration
  are involved?

- Are they able to deliver what is needed in the timescale required?

- Is training an ongoing requirement and are the financial implications known?

- Will the organization commit itself to the cost of acquiring the services of a high quality training and development manager?

Action Check 31

Training and management – How will skills be developed?

Managers are central to introducing effective change in any organization. They must have ownership of the changes and the ability and motivation to deliver them. Firstly, stop all extraneous management training that is not focused on what the organization needs. This saves money and buys time to reinvest in training packages which are properly thought through and which add value to the organization and not just to the individual.

♦ Identify the managerial skills/performance criteria required by your organization over the next five years, at each managerial level.

♦ Identify good performance by either using a series of focus groups or by identifying what good performance looks like in your organization by looking at high performers.

♦ Can the information gained above be used to design a series of development workshops which focus both on auditing your current managerial stock against your organizational requirements and on identifying individuals' development needs?

♦ Identify and train internal assessors for development workshops. Can assessors from outside the organization be brought in? Will they bring an independent perspective and a fresh pair of eyes to the situation? Can they distinguish the wood from the trees?

♦ Can development workshops be run over two to three days? Will emphasis be on individuals and confidentiality? Will attendance be voluntary or compulsory?

- Will the results of the development workshops be fed back to the Board?

- Can the results be anonymized? Should they be?

Action Check 32

*Training and management
– How are managers
developed?*

Development workshops are likely to identify three broad groups; high flyers, moderate to good managers, moderate to poor performers. The first two groups will be worth investing in. Ensure there are good organizationally based development pro-grammes focusing on improving their skills and competencies. Members of the third group should probably never have been appointed as managers in the first place. Is further investment in them worthwhile? Work with them on an individual basis to find the way forward. Beware! You may have to take some difficult decisions!

♦ How will the organization deal with poorly functioning managers?

♦ Will the Board agree to redundancy packages?

- ♦ Is there a case for disciplinary action?

- ♦ Are managers sufficiently knowledgeable and trained in disciplinary issues?

Action Check 33

Manpower information

Can manpower information be used as a management tool?

What manpower information is available to the Board, managers and others? Staff turnover, absence ratios, overtime and agency working, study leave and a host of other indicators make up the cost equation of the largest part of the budget. The Board will need to have regular access to information in a style that it can understand to enable it to identify trends and initiate action.

♦ What information will the Board need and how often will they need it?

♦ How will the information be presented? Modern computer software can make the most indigestible information interesting.

♦ How will progress be monitored and performance improved?

♦ How will the outcomes be measured?

♦ Do some departments work a disproportionate amount of overtime? Can this be linked to one manager or one department?

Action Check 34

Induction

Is there a 'getting started' or induction programme?

The memory of how they are treated during their first few days in an organization will remain with new staff for the rest of the time they work with the organization.

◆ Are new staff made to feel welcome? How?

◆ What form does induction take?

◆ Is there a specific induction course/programme?

- What is included on the course? Is it relevant?

- Will new staff (regardless of seniority) meet key, senior staff including members of the Board?

- How will new members of staff be involved in the organization's goals and objectives?

- Will new staff have a role to play in reviewing the goals?

- If the organization occupies a complicated campus, how will new members of the staff familiarize themselves with the geography?

♦ How welcoming is the organization to new staff?

♦ If new staff are to live-in and are expected to arrive on their first day at a weekend or out of hours, who will be on hand to welcome them? Will they have enough simple supplies such as coffee, milk, etc? Will there be a welcome pack for them?

♦ How will the success of the induction programme be evaluated?

♦ Will younger members of staff, perhaps away from home for the first time, have a mentor to chaperone them during their first few days?

Action Check 35

Recruitment

Does the recruitment policy work?

Recruitment is costly. Employing the right staff starts with good interviewing techniques, and that means training for any member of staff with a responsibility for recruitment. Of more strategic importance is the source of new recruits. New people joining the organization from other parts of the country may need assistance with housing and other welfare considerations. Local recruitment has fewer hidden costs. Once staff are recruited to the organization, what makes them stay?

♦ Does the organization have a recruitment strategy?

♦ Is the recruitment strategy and the staff selection process based on a clear understanding of what constitutes good performance?

◆ How can you ensure only good performers are recruited?

◆ Does the recruitment strategy complement the strategic needs of the organization?

◆ What resources will be applied to getting staff trained in interviewing techniques?

◆ Is there a review of how successful the recruitment process is? Do good people get away?

◆ How easy is it to join the organization? Does it involve waiting for interviews, and wading through mountains of paper? Is the process hostile or helpful?

Action Check 36

Retention

Will good staff stay?

Why do staff leave? Properly constructed exit interviews, conducted by a neutral person, can provide useful data and an insight into why staff leave. If themes emerge from the interviews, policies can be shaped to deal with the wastage of staff and the costs of replacing them.

- ◆ What is the staff turnover rate?

- ◆ Are there seasonal fluctuations?

- ◆ Is age an issue?

♦ As a percentage of the organization's working population, is there a higher turnover in identifiable groups?

♦ Will exit interviews be carried out for all staff?

♦ Who will conduct the interview?

♦ Will the results be treated in confidence and data rendered anonymous?

♦ Will the Board receive a summary of the outcome data on exit interviews?

- ◆ Will any attempt be made to keep in touch with leavers, in the hope that they may wish to return at some future date?

Action Check 37

Discipline

Is the organization well disciplined?

Generally, staff like to work in an atmosphere of efficiency, where discipline is seen to be fair and management are not afraid to act in the interests of staff and patients. Incidents of poor discipline are often indicators of the morale and functioning of the organization.

- ◆ Does the Board monitor disciplinary issues?

- ◆ How often are disciplinary rules reviewed? How are the results communicated to the staff?

- ◆ Is there a pattern of poor discipline?

◆ Are certain disciplinary offences common and do they repeat themselves?

◆ Can conclusions be drawn about management skills from discipline within the organization?

◆ Does the organization have a clear set of disciplinary rules?

◆ Are the rules published and do members of staff have their own copies of them?

◆ Does the organization have a disciplinary procedure which is fair and facilitates effective and timely action?

♦ Is the disciplinary procedure published and do members of staff each have a copy?

♦ Are disciplinary appeal hearings conducted swiftly, efficiently and fairly?

♦ Are Board directors available, at short notice, to hear appeals promptly?

♦ Is the staff-side adequately resourced to represent staff properly?

♦ Are managers properly trained to deal with staff fairly, consistently and with understanding?

• Do the same names keep appearing, either as defendants or accusers?

• Are appeal decisions consistent?

• What is the organization's record of success with industrial tribunals?

• Does the organization have sufficient resources and training to deal with industrial tribunals? Does the organization engage the services of solicitors? How is their performance measured?

Action Check 38

Equal opportunities

Will the organization be an equal opportunity employer?

Becoming an equal opportunity employer may require a radical rethink about recruitment techniques, promotion, dismissal and virtually every other aspect of the work of the personnel department!

- ◆ Will the Board want to develop an equal opportunity strategy?

- ◆ Is the Board aware of the cost implications?

- ◆ Can the Board see the benefits?

- Does the Board understand other implications?

- Will the commitment to being an equal opportunity employer bring about improvements in the organization?

- Can the improvements be measured?

Action Check 39

Employing women

Is the organization an easy place for women to work in?

Nearly 80 percent of hands-on healthcare is delivered by women, yet fewer than 12 percent become senior managers. Over half the students entering medical school are women, but fewer than three percent become consultant surgeons. Is something wrong?

♦ Is it easy for women to join the organization?

♦ Is it easy for women to work in the organization?

♦ Are meetings held at times which conflict with family commitments? Do meetings have to be held at these times?

♦ Is the organization a safe place for women to work?

♦ Is the campus well lit; are staff car parks remote from the main buildings?

♦ Does the organization keep in touch with leavers?

♦ Are leavers offered refresher courses, to update their skills, regardless of whether they have announced a return to work or not?

- Is it easy to return to work?

- How many jobshare posts are there in the organization?

- Is child care an issue?

- Does the organization have a register of child minders?

- Can the organization facilitate a self-help group to enable parents to get together?

- ♦ How good are the creche facilities, are they open at the right times and are they affordable?

- ♦ How flexible are contract arrangements?

Action Check 40

AIDS and HIV

What should the organization do about AIDS and HIV?

The possibility of medical staff contracting HIV and the impact that can have on patients and staff is likely to be an increasingly difficult issue.

♦ Have all staff at risk been advised of Department of Health guidance?

♦ Is there a local policy?

♦ If a member of staff reports that they are HIV positive, does the organization have a prepared response?

♦ How will the organization handle any press enquiries which may arise?

♦ How will patients be contacted?

♦ Who will offer counselling to patients?

♦ Where will the staff come from to handle telephone en-quiries?

♦ When will they be trained?

♦ How will the privacy of the member of staff be protected?

♦ How will the member of staff be supported?

♦ How can the organization create an atmosphere of confidence in which sufferers can feel able to make an early declaration?

Action Check 41

Hepatitis B

Should the organization consider the risks to staff of Hepatitis B?
In some services there is a significant risk to staff from Hepatitis B. Should the Board consider the risk and make provision to protect staff.

♦ Do you have a local policy concerning Hepatitis B?

♦ Has the organization evaluated the risk of Hepatitis B?

♦ Should the issue be raised with the staff?

♦ Should the organization offer a voluntary programme of inoculation?

♦ Can an inoculation programme be funded by the organization?

♦ Should the responsibility for taking precautions rest with individuals? Who should make their own provision?

♦ Should new staff be treated differently from existing members of staff?

SECTION 3

MEASURING SUCCESS

Action Check 42

Success

What are the HR success factors?

Much depends on the HR team. How will the organization measure the success of its HR policies? Is the HR team seen as a service provider for the rest of the organization? Is it possible to draw up a service specification to reflect a service style relationship? Could the HR team provide a service in an internal market, tested from time to time against outside competition?

♦ What is the percentage of staff who consistently achieve individual goal/s and targets year after year? Does this reveal where development work is needed?

♦ Has the organization consistently achieved its business plan goals year after year?

- How many staff have transferred to the local pay scheme?

- Are staff turnover levels down?

- Is the organization a healthier place? Is sickness absence down?

- What is the pay bill? What are the trends?

- What is the staff cost per patient treated? Are there any trends?

- What can be deduced from levels of trade union member-ship? Do more members mean that the staff feel threatened; do fewer members mean staff feel confident, or is membership based on the prowess and popularity of local organizers?

- Are contracts with commissioners delivered and renewed as new contracts?

- What is the outcome of staff/customer feedback question-naires?

- Is the organization well disciplined? Are there fewer or more hearings and appeals? What are the outcomes? What are the trends?

♦ What is the cost of the HR function as a percentage of the total budget? Can any trends be detected?

♦ Can the effectiveness of the management development programme and its contribution to success be evaluated?

Index

absenteeism, due to sickness
53–5, 116
accountability for payroll
failures 58
accuracy, payroll data 32,
58–60
age profile of staff 34
turnover 95
agency nursing 51
and pay remodelling 39
AIDS 108–10
annual leave 56
annual uplifts in pay 49
appeals, disciplinary 100, 101
arbitration facilities 29–30
attitude surveys 11

bandings, pay spine 41–6
bank arrangements 51–2
bank holiday rates 57
bonuses 48
business plans 7–9
business strategy 7–9

chaperones 92
child care 106–7
commitment
of managers 17–18
to training 75
competitors 49

computers 88
conciliation facilities 29
conferences 76–7
consultants 61
contracts, employment 35, 107
costs
human resources 118
locum 52
overtime 51
pay remodelling 38–9
payroll 59
training 75–6, 82
counselling, patients with
HIV/AIDS 109
crèche facilities 107
culture
departmental 20
organizational 10–11
customer service training 60

design, jobs 63–5
development workshops
84–5, 86
directors
executive 21
nonexecutive 28
disagreements with trade
unions 29
discipline
evaluation 117

organizational   98–101
of poor managers   87
of sick leave takers   55
discussions with trade unions
   28
doctors   50

education and training   75–7
   attitudes towards   10
   for HIV/AIDS enquiries   109
   in-house   78–9
   payroll staff   60
   performance management
      67, 71
   for recruitment   93, 94
   reengineering management
      80
   reprofiling   65
   restructuring   81–2
   skills development   83–7
   of trade unionists   28
employment
   contracts   35, 107
equal opportunities   102–3
evaluation
   job   36, 37–8
      pay spines   41
   performance   67, 84
   performance management
      schemes   72
   recruitment
      programmes   94
   of success   115–18
   training   76, 79
executive directors   21
exit interviews   95, 96

finance department   19, 20–1
fixed allowances   48
flexibility, employment
   contracts   35, 107

freedom, Trust   16
full-time staff   35

Hepatitis B   111–12
HIV   108–10
hours, working   56

incentives
   pay as   15, 48
   savings as   62
individual performance   66–9
induction programmes   90–2
industrial tribunals   101
in-house training   78–9
inoculation programmes,
   Hepatitis B   112
internal bank arrangements
   51–2
interviews
   exit   95, 96
   recruitment   93, 94

job evaluation   36, 37–8
   pay spines   41
job opportunities   62
job satisfaction   63
job sharing   35, 106

language, Mission and Values
   statements   6
leaders, team   20
league tables, sickness   54
leave
   annual   56
   sickness   53–5
legally binding agreements   30
locum costs   52

managers
   commitment   17–18
   development   86–7

discipline 87, 100
pay remodelling 50
performance management
     70, 71
performance reviews 67
restructuring 80–2
skills development 83–5
welfare visits 54
manpower information 88–9
medical certificates 55
meetings
timing, and women 105
with trade unions 27, 28–9
mentors 92
merit awards 50
Mission and Values
statements 5–6
monitoring, performance
management 67
multiple table bargaining 27

new staff, induction 90–2
night duty payments 57
nonexecutive directors 28

occupational health service
     54, 55
open book approach 29
opportunities, job 62
organizational values 5–6
overtime 51–2
distribution 89
and pay remodelling 39

part-time staff 35
pay 15
annual uplifts 49
attitudes towards 10
bank rates 52
bargaining 25–7
freedom 16

managerial commitment 17
modelling 31–2
options 23–4
performance management
     69
performance related 47–8
dangers 50
pay spines 42, 43
remodelling 36–40
dangers 50
spines 40, 41–6
teamwork 19–22
payroll accuracy 32, 58–60
pendulum arbitration 30
performance management
     70–2
commitment to 50
individuals 66–9
productivity issues 73–4
performance related pay 47–8
dangers 50
pay spines 42, 43
productivity 73–4

recognition of trade unions
     35–30
recruitment 34, 95–7
job design 64
redundancy packages 86
refresher courses 105
representation of staff, in
disciplinary actions 100
see also trade unions
reprofiling 61–5
resources for patients 10
retention, staff 64, 95–7
reviews
performance 67
skill mix 61
productivity 74
rewards

executive directors   21
freedom   16
see also pay
rules, disciplinary   99

safety, organizational   105
salaries *see* pay
satisfaction, job   63
savings
  for pay remodelling   39
  from reprofiling   62
seasonal fluctuations, staff
  turnover   95
shift payments   57
sickness, staff   34, 53–5, 116
single table bargaining   27
skill mix
  job design   64–5
  reviews   61
    productivity   74
skills development   83–5
solicitors   101
staff
  age profile   34
  attitudes   10–11
  employment contracts   35
  induction   90–2
  job design   63–5
  Mission and Values
    statement   5
  pay spines   40
  recruitment   34, 64, 93–4
  representation *see* trade
    unions
  reprofiling   61–2
  sickness   34, 53–5, 116
  turnover   33, 64, 95–7, 116
staff organizations
  bank rates of pay   52
  recognition of   25, 27
statutory days, payment   57

strategy, business   7–9
success measurement   115–18
surveys, of attitudes   10–11

teamworking   19–22
  performance management
    66
technology   64
trade unions
  annual uplift in pay   49
  job evaluation   38
  membership   117
  pay remodelling   50
  recognition of   25–30
training *see* education and
  training
training departments   76
Transfer of Undertaking
  (Protection of Employment)
  Regulations   36
tribunals, industrial   101
turnover, staff   33, 95–7, 116
  job design   64

unit labour costs   73

values statements   5–6

wages *see* pay
weekend rates   57
welfare visits   54
'Whitley' pay scales
  and alternatives   23
  annual uplifts   49
  complexity   50
  job evaluation   37
  pay spines   40, 44
women   104–7
  job design   64
working hours   56